PALEO PASTA

Gluten-Free Pasta Recipes for a Paleo Diet

By John Chatham

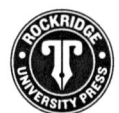

ISBN: Print 978-1-62315-107-2 | eBook 978-1-62315-108-9

CONTENTS

Chapter 2: Paleo Pasta Sauce and Noodles

Chapter 3: Paleo Baked Pastas

INTRODUCTION

Spaghetti with meatballs, linguine with clams, fettuccini alfredo, macaroni and cheese—if you're like many Western eaters, these childhood comfort foods have been dietary staples since you were barely old enough to chew. Pasta plays such an integral role in our lives: kids eagerly slurp it down, athletes carb-load on it before a big event, and families gather in kitchens to create favorite dishes together, making memories that last a lifetime. But now you've decided to pursue the Paleo lifestyle, which absolutely forbids traditional pasta. Fortunately, we refuse to accept that these luscious dishes are a thing of the past!

When Dr. Walter L. Voegtlin created the Paleo diet in 1975, it was a somewhat radical path to a healthy, disease-free existence. It required giving up all breads, grains, pasta, many root vegetables, and all refined foods. Basically, to truly eat caveman-style, you'd have to walk away from the Western diet and every culinary temptation you face simply walking down the street every day. One of the biggest temptations, of course, is pasta and many of the decadent sauces that accompany it.

As difficult as it may sound, finding substitutes for many foods is fairly easy as long as you possess a modicum of creativity and a willingness to try new things. The tricky part is re-creating such foods as pastas, because traditional versions are dependent upon gluten, a protein found in wheat flour that lends structure and is responsible for that soft, elastic texture we love. Without it, your breads and pastas will be crumbly and dense; with it, your foods aren't Paleo friendly and may also cause digestive upset and disease.

Nevertheless, rather than accept a life without pasta, you'll find there exists a multitude of alternatives, and this collection offers you a broad range of gluten-free recipes for homemade pastas both delicious and nutritious. The following pages present a wide variety of favorite recipes for delicate, tasty, Paleo pastas you're sure to love. And since pasta alone simply won't do, it's accompanied by a tempting selection of Paleo and gluten-free sauces to top it off. It was great fun creating these delectable dishes, and eating them should be even more so . . . *mangia bene*!

SECTION ONE
Gluten-Free Paleo Pasta

- **Chapter 1:**   Homemade Paleo Noodles

- **Chapter 2:**   Paleo Pasta Sauce and Noodles

- **Chapter 3:**   Paleo Baked Pastas

HOMEMADE PALEO NOODLES

Paleo Pasta Dough

Homemade pasta is a special treat and it's often found in first-rate Italian restaurants, but it remains a strict no-no on the Paleo diet. While there are plenty of packaged Paleo-friendly noodles, if you're a pasta lover, you may still crave some fresh noodles, and this recipe fits the bill. Ground flax gives this dough a hearty, wheat-like flavor, but without the carbs and gluten. It's easy to prepare and will stand up to your favorite marinara sauce well. If you'd like it to have a lighter color, use golden flaxseed instead.

- 3½ cups ground flaxseed, divided
- ½ cup warm water
- 2 large eggs
- 2 teaspoons sea salt
- 6 tablespoons coconut flour
- ½ cup arrowroot starch, plus more for kneading

Combine ½ cup flaxseed with ½ cup warm water. Stir and add the eggs and salt. Set aside.

In a large bowl, combine the remaining flaxseed with the coconut flour and arrowroot starch. Stir to combine.

Add the wet flax mixture to the dry ingredients, and stir with a wooden spoon until you have a slightly sticky but firm dough. If the dough is too wet, add some more arrowroot.

Knead the dough for about 5 minutes until it is smooth and slightly elastic to the touch.

Roll out the dough using a standard pasta maker, adding more arrowroot if necessary. Cut it into strips, or use flat sheets for lasagna or ravioli.

When you are ready to use the pasta, cook it in boiling water for about 20–30 seconds, depending on the size of the noodle. Strain and serve with your favorite sauce.

For best results, cook and eat all the pasta as soon as it is prepared.

Serves 4.

Fresh Spinach Pasta

This fresh pasta made from ground flaxseed includes a hefty dose of spinach, which will lightly flavor your favorite pasta dish. To get the most out of the delicate flavor, eat this with a simple sauce or just plain with some melted butter. If you don't have a pasta machine, you can roll it out between two sheets of parchment paper, though producing a thin noodle with this method won't be easy.

- 6 cups fresh spinach leaves, stemmed
- 3½ cups ground flaxseed, divided
- ¼ cup warm water
- 2 large eggs
- 2 teaspoons sea salt
- 6 tablespoons coconut flour
- ½ cup arrowroot starch, plus more for kneading

Bring a pot of water to a boil. Add the spinach and cook for about 3 minutes. Drain well and lay on paper towels. Squeeze as much of the liquid out as you can. Finely chop the spinach either in a food processor or by hand.

Combine ½ cup flaxseed with ¼ cup warm water. Stir and add the eggs, salt, and chopped spinach. Stir until well combined.

In a large bowl, combine the remaining flaxseed with the coconut flour and arrowroot starch. Stir to combine.

Add the spinach mixture to the dry ingredients, and stir with a wooden spoon until you have a slightly sticky but firm dough. If the dough is too wet, add some more arrowroot.

Knead the dough for about 5 minutes until it is smooth and slightly elastic to the touch.

Roll out the dough using a standard pasta maker, adding more arrowroot if necessary. Cut it into strips, or use flat sheets for lasagna or ravioli.

When you are ready to use the pasta, cook it in boiling water for about 20–30 seconds, depending on the size of the noodle. Strain and serve with your favorite sauce.

For best results, cook and eat all the pasta as soon as it's prepared.

Serves 4.

Mushroom Pasta

This earthy and flavorful pasta pairs beautifully with a hearty marinara or even a delicate butter sauce. It's delicious served plain with a pat of butter as well. While the recipe calls for button mushrooms, feel free to use any variety you like. You'll be surprised at how much the flavor varies depending on the type of mushrooms you choose. Be sure to use fresh mushrooms for best results.

- 2 tablespoons grass-fed butter
- 2 cups button mushrooms, sliced
- 3½ cups ground flaxseed, divided
- ¼ cup warm water
- 2 large eggs
- 2 teaspoons sea salt
- 6 tablespoons coconut flour
- ½ cup arrowroot starch, plus more for kneading

Heat the butter in a large skillet over medium-high heat. Add the mushrooms and sauté until golden brown. Allow the mushrooms to cool for a few minutes, and transfer to a food processor. Pulse until very finely chopped but not a paste.

Combine ½ cup flaxseed with ¼ cup warm water. Stir and add the eggs and salt. Add the mushroom mixture and mix well.

In a large bowl, combine the remaining flaxseed with the coconut flour and arrowroot starch. Stir to combine.

Add the mushroom mixture to the dry ingredients, and stir with a wooden spoon until you have a slightly sticky but firm dough. If the dough is too wet, add some more arrowroot.

Knead the dough for about 5 minutes until it is smooth and slightly elastic to the touch.

Roll out the dough using a standard pasta maker, adding more arrowroot if necessary. Cut it into strips, or use flat sheets for lasagna or ravioli.

When you are ready to use the pasta, cook it in boiling water for about 20–30 seconds, depending on the size of the noodle. Strain and serve with your favorite sauce.

For best results, cook and eat all the pasta as soon as it's prepared.

Serves 4.

Fresh Herb Pasta

You can customize this fresh pasta dough using whatever herbs you have available. Rosemary, thyme, and oregano make a good choice, or if you're serving it with a Mediterranean dish, some fresh mint is nice, too. Fresh herbs are best, but dried can be used in a pinch—simply use half the amount. For an additional burst of fresh flavor, add the zest of a lemon to the pasta as well. Serve this with a lighter sauce for best results.

- 3½ cups ground flaxseed, divided
- ½ cup warm water
- 2 large eggs
- 2 teaspoons sea salt
- ½ cup fresh herbs of your choice, finely chopped
- 6 tablespoons coconut flour
- ½ cup arrowroot starch

Combine ½ cup flaxseed with ½ cup warm water. Stir and add the eggs and salt. Set aside.

In a large bowl, combine the remaining flaxseed with the herbs, coconut flour, and arrowroot starch. Stir to combine, being careful with delicate herbs.

Add the wet flax mixture to the dry ingredients, and stir with a wooden spoon until you have a slightly sticky but firm dough. If the dough is too wet, add some more arrowroot.

Knead the dough for about 5 minutes until it is smooth and slightly elastic to the touch.

Roll out the dough using a standard pasta maker, adding more arrowroot if necessary. Cut it into strips, or use flat sheets for lasagna or ravioli.

When you are ready to use the pasta, cook it in boiling water for about 20–30 seconds, depending on the size of the noodle. Strain and serve with your favorite sauce.

For best results, cook and eat all the pasta as soon as it's prepared.

Serves 4.

Roasted Red Pepper Pasta

Like many flavored pastas, this bright orange pasta is best served with a light sauce to maximize its flavor. To save some time, skip the step of roasting the peppers and use your favorite jarred variety. For a little heat, add a jalapeño to the mix.

- 2 large red bell peppers
- 1 tablespoon olive oil
- 3½ cups ground flaxseed, divided
- 2 large eggs
- 2 teaspoons sea salt
- 6 tablespoons coconut flour
- ½ cup arrowroot starch

Cut the tops off the peppers, and remove the seeds and membranes. Slice the peppers in order to open them up and lay them flat on a sheet pan. Preheat broiler to high, and broil them for 5–10 minutes until the skins are blackened. Remove from the oven, and place the peppers in a paper bag for 15 minutes.

Remove peppers from the bag, and transfer to a food processor with the olive oil. Puree until smooth.

Combine ½ cup flaxseed with the pureed peppers in a medium bowl. Stir and add the eggs and salt. Set aside.

In a large bowl, combine the remaining flaxseed with the coconut flour and arrowroot starch. Stir to combine.

Add the pepper mixture to the dry ingredients, and stir with a wooden spoon until you have a slightly sticky, but firm dough. If the dough is too wet, add some more arrowroot.

Knead the dough for about 5 minutes until it is smooth and slightly elastic to the touch.

Roll out the dough using a standard pasta maker, adding more arrowroot if necessary. Cut it into strips, or use flat sheets for lasagna or ravioli.

When you are ready to use the pasta, cook it in boiling water for about 20–30 seconds, depending on the size of the noodle. Strain and serve with your favorite sauce.

For best results, cook and eat all the pasta as soon as it's prepared.

Serves 4.

Roasted Garlic Pasta

While the amount of garlic called for here might seem like a lot, don't be tempted to leave some out for fear of it being too strong. Roasting garlic turns the normally pungent and spicy flavor mellow and aromatic, so the end result is a delicious fresh pasta dish with your favorite marinara or some shrimp sautéed in butter.

- 2 heads of garlic
- 1 tablespoon olive oil
- 3½ cups ground flaxseed, divided
- ¼ cup warm water
- 2 large eggs
- 2 teaspoons sea salt
- 6 tablespoons coconut flour
- ½ cup arrowroot starch

Preheat oven to 400 degrees F.

Slice the stem end of each of the garlic bulbs, and lay them on a piece of foil, cut side up. Drizzle with the olive oil, and seal the foil tightly.

Bake for about 45 minutes, remove from oven, and carefully open the packet.

When the garlic is slightly cool, squeeze the browned cloves into a small bowl, and mash well with a fork.

Combine ½ cup flaxseed with ¼ cup warm water. Stir in the garlic, and add the eggs and salt. Set aside.

In a large bowl, combine the remaining flaxseed with the coconut flour and arrowroot starch. Stir to combine.

Add the garlic mixture to the dry ingredients, and stir with a wooden spoon until you have a slightly sticky but firm dough. If the dough is too wet, add some more arrowroot.

Knead the dough for about 5 minutes until it is smooth and slightly elastic to the touch.

Roll out the dough using a standard pasta maker, adding more arrowroot if necessary. Cut it into strips, or use flat sheets for lasagna or ravioli.

When you are ready to use the pasta, cook it in boiling water for about 20–30 seconds, depending on the size of the noodle. Strain and serve with your favorite sauce.

For best results, cook and eat all the pasta as soon as it's prepared.

Serves 4.

Sun-Dried Tomato Basil Pasta

Sun-dried tomatoes and fresh basil make this pasta extra flavorful. It's perfect to eat in the summer with some fresh, lightly sautéed vegetables and herbs. It's also quite appealing with a light marinara sauce.

- 3½ cups ground flaxseed, divided
- ½ cup warm water
- 2 large eggs
- 2 teaspoons sea salt
- ½ cup sun-dried tomatoes, minced
- 1 bunch basil leaves, minced
- 6 tablespoons coconut flour
- ½ cup arrowroot starch

Combine ½ cup flaxseed with ½ cup warm water. Stir and add the eggs and salt. Set aside.

In a large bowl, combine the remaining flaxseed with the sun-dried tomatoes, basil, coconut flour, and arrowroot starch. Stir to combine.

Add the wet flax mixture to the dry ingredients, and stir with a wooden spoon until you have a slightly sticky but firm dough. If the dough is too wet, add some more arrowroot.

Knead the dough for about 5 minutes until it is smooth and slightly elastic to the touch.

Roll out the dough using a standard pasta maker, adding more arrowroot if necessary. Cut it into strips, or use flat sheets for lasagna or ravioli.

When you are ready to use the pasta, cook it in boiling water for about 20–30 seconds, depending on the size of the noodle. Strain and serve with your favorite sauce.

For best results, cook and eat all the pasta as soon as it's prepared.

Serves 4.

Roasted Beet Pasta

This bright pink pasta is a unique dish to serve to guests, and it will surely have everyone talking. It's got a light, earthy flavor that is perfect in a pasta salad tossed with some orange segments and chopped walnuts. You can also enjoy it plain or tossed with some grass-fed butter as a brightly colored side dish. For variation, try making this with golden beets, which will give you a bright yellow noodle.

• 1 large beet	• 2 large eggs
• 1 teaspoon olive oil	• 2 teaspoons sea salt
• 3½ cups ground golden flaxseed, divided	• 6 tablespoons coconut flour
	• ½ cup arrowroot starch

Preheat oven to 400 degrees F.

Slice both ends off the beet, and lay it on a sheet of foil. Drizzle with olive oil, and seal the foil. Roast for 45 minutes.

Remove the beet from the oven, and carefully open the foil. Allow to cool, then remove the skin.

Place the beet in a food processor, and puree until smooth.

Combine ½ cup flaxseed with the pureed beet in a medium bowl. Stir and add the eggs and salt. Set aside.

In a large bowl, combine the remaining flaxseed with the coconut flour and arrowroot starch. Stir to combine.

Add the beet mixture to the dry ingredients, and stir with a wooden spoon until you have a slightly sticky but firm dough. If the dough is too wet, add some more arrowroot.

Knead the dough for about 5 minutes until it is smooth and slightly elastic to the touch.

Roll out the dough using a standard pasta maker, adding more arrowroot if necessary. Cut it into strips, or use flat sheets for lasagna or ravioli.

When you are ready to use the pasta, cook it in boiling water for about 20–30 seconds, depending on the size of the noodle. Strain and serve with your favorite sauce.

For best results, cook and eat all the pasta as soon as it's prepared.

Serves 4.

Lemon Pepper Pasta

This delightfully peppery, fresh pasta is delicious with sautéed shrimp or chicken. Add some fresh vegetables, and you've got an easy and flavorful meal. You may be tempted to use a prepared lemon pepper mix—skip this, as many seasonings contain additives and preservatives that don't adhere to the Paleo diet.

- 3½ cups ground flaxseed, divided
- ¼ cup warm water
- Juice of 1 lemon
- 2 large eggs
- 2 teaspoons sea salt
- Zest of 1 lemon
- 2 teaspoons freshly ground black pepper
- 6 tablespoons coconut flour
- ½ cup arrowroot starch

Combine ½ cup flaxseed with ¼ cup warm water and the lemon juice. Stir and add the eggs and salt. Set aside.

In a large bowl, combine the remaining flaxseed with the lemon zest, pepper, coconut flour, and arrowroot starch. Stir to combine.

Add the wet flax mixture to the dry ingredients, and stir with a wooden spoon until you have a slightly sticky, but firm dough. If the dough is too wet, add some more arrowroot.

Knead the dough for about 5 minutes until it is smooth and slightly elastic to the touch.

Roll out the dough using a standard pasta maker, adding more arrowroot if necessary. Cut it into strips, or use flat sheets for lasagna or ravioli.

When you are ready to use the pasta, cook it in boiling water for about 20–30 seconds, depending on the size of the noodle. Strain and serve with your favorite sauce.

For best results, cook and eat all the pasta as soon as it's prepared.

Serves 4.

Chili Lime Pasta

This Southwestern-spiced pasta is great with some grilled chicken and fresh cilantro. It also works particularly well with an avocado cream sauce, as the spiciness of the chili pepper cuts right through the mild avocado cream. Feel free to add more or less crushed red pepper flakes to the dough, depending on how spicy you like it—the teaspoon called for here will give you subtle but flavorful pasta that is not terribly hot.

- 3½ cups ground flaxseed, divided
- ½ cup warm water
- Juice of 2 limes
- 2 large eggs
- 2 teaspoons sea salt
- Zest of 2 limes
- 1 teaspoon red pepper flakes, crushed
- 6 tablespoons coconut flour
- ½ cup arrowroot starch

Combine ½ cup flaxseed with the water and lime juice. Stir and add the eggs and salt. Set aside.

In a large bowl, combine the remaining flaxseed with the lime zest, crushed red pepper flakes, coconut flour, and arrowroot starch. Stir to combine.

Add the wet flax mixture to the dry ingredients, and stir with a wooden spoon until you have a slightly sticky but firm dough. If the dough is too wet, add some more arrowroot.

Knead the dough for about 5 minutes until it is smooth and slightly elastic to the touch.

Roll out the dough using a standard pasta maker, adding more arrowroot if necessary. Cut it into strips, or use flat sheets for lasagna or ravioli.

When you are ready to use the pasta, cook it in boiling water for about 20–30 seconds, depending on the size of the noodle. Strain and serve with your favorite sauce.

For best results, cook and eat all the pasta as soon as it's prepared.

Serves 4.

Kalamata Olive Pasta

This savory pasta is well suited for Mediterranean dishes but tastes fantastic paired with your favorite tomato-based sauce as well. Feel free to substitute your preferred variety for the kalamata olives, or use an assortment for interest.

- 3½ cups ground flaxseed, divided
- ½ cup warm water
- 2 large eggs
- 2 teaspoons sea salt
- ½ cup kalamata olives, pitted and finely chopped
- 6 tablespoons coconut flour
- ½ cup arrowroot starch, plus more for kneading

Combine ½ cup flaxseed with ½ cup warm water. Stir and add the eggs and salt. Set aside.

In a large bowl, combine the remaining flaxseed with the chopped olives, coconut flour, and arrowroot starch. Stir to combine.

Add the wet flax mixture to the dry ingredients, and stir with a wooden spoon until you have a slightly sticky but firm dough. If the dough is too wet, add some more arrowroot.

Knead the dough for about 5 minutes until it is smooth and slightly elastic to the touch.

Roll out the dough using a standard pasta maker, adding more arrowroot if necessary. Cut it into strips, or use flat sheets for lasagna or ravioli.

When you are ready to use the pasta, cook it in boiling water for about 20–30 seconds, depending on the size of the noodle. Strain and serve with your favorite sauce.

For best results, cook and eat all the pasta as soon as it's prepared.

Serves 4.

Sweet Potato Gnocchi

These delicious and tender gnocchi are made with sweet potatoes instead of the traditional, starchy, white variety, but that doesn't make them any less delicious—if anything, their flavor is enhanced. You can serve these with your preferred marinara sauce, but they are also fabulous with some browned, grass-fed butter with crispy sage leaves. Experiment, and you are sure to discover some favorite combinations of your own!

- 2 medium sweet potatoes
- 1 large egg
- 2 cups almond flour

Preheat oven to 400 degrees F.

Bake the sweet potatoes for 1 hour, or until tender when pierced with a fork. Remove from oven and allow to cool completely.

Scoop the flesh from the sweet potatoes, and mash them until completely smooth, either by hand or using a mixer. Refrigerate the mixture for 30 minutes.

Remove from the refrigerator, and add the egg. Stir well and slowly add the almond flour about ½ cup at a time, until you have a stiff dough.

To make the gnocchi, divide the dough into 3 or 4 pieces, rolling each into a long rope, about the thickness of your thumb.

Using a sharp knife, cut each rope into ½-inch pieces. If desired, use a fork to make the classic gnocchi imprint on each one.

To cook, bring a large pot of water to a boil. Add the gnocchi and cook until they begin to float to the top. Drain and serve immediately with your desired sauce or toppings.

Serves 4.

PALEO PASTA SAUCE AND NOODLES

Creamy Paleo Fettuccini

This deliciously creamy pasta dish gets its creaminess and flavor from a ripened avocado. You can serve this alone or with grilled and sliced chicken breast for a meal reminiscent of your favorite Italian restaurant, but without the carbs. Feel free to use any flavor of fresh pasta you'd like, as this sauce complements almost any variety. Since you are reheating the pasta in the sauce, it's especially important you don't overcook it, or you'll end up with extra-mushy pasta.

- 1 ripe avocado, peeled and pitted
- Juice of 1 lemon
- 1 garlic clove, smashed
- 2 tablespoons olive oil
- 1 recipe Paleo Pasta Dough, cut into fettuccini noodles

Put the avocado, lemon, and garlic in the bowl of a food processor. Puree until smooth and slowly drizzle in the olive oil. Transfer the sauce to a deep skillet, and turn on low heat.

Bring a large pot of salted water to a boil, and add the pasta. Cook for about 20 seconds and drain, being careful not to overcook.

Add the pasta to the skillet with the sauce and toss. Serve immediately.

Serves 4.

Paleo Spaghetti and Marinara

There are many brands of Paleo-diet-approved pasta on the market these days, and while some are OK, many are full of the same processed ingredients you might be trying to avoid. This version uses a surprise ingredient that is actually quite delicious: zucchini noodles. A spiral slicer makes cutting the squash into noodles a cinch, but a veggie peeler or mandolin slicer will do. You can try to use a sharp knife, but your results may vary. The sauce is extremely easy to prepare, and you'll be amazed that anyone would spend all day making a pot of sauce after you taste this version. If you can find San Marzano tomatoes, buy them—they make this sauce extra special.

For the sauce:

- 2 (32-ounce) cans whole tomatoes, preferably San Marzano
- 2 tablespoons grass-fed butter
- ¼ small onion, in one piece

For the noodles:

- 2 tablespoons olive oil
- 2 medium zucchini, cut into noodles using a spiral slicer or the julienne blade on a mandolin

Make the sauce:

Combine the tomatoes, butter, and onion in a large saucepot. Bring to a boil and reduce heat. Simmer for 45 minutes until the tomatoes are broken down. For a smoother sauce, puree in a blender or food processor.

Cook the noodles:

In a large skillet, heat the olive oil over medium heat. Add the zucchini noodles, and toss until just heated through—don't overcook. Pour the sauce over the noodles, and stir to combine. Serve hot.

If you have leftover sauce, you can store it in the refrigerator for up to 3 days. The zucchini noodles should be eaten right away.

Serves 4.

Spinach and Mushroom Ravioli with Dairy-Free Pesto

These simple-to-prepare ravioli come to life with a deliciously flavorful pesto sauce. If you have ravioli cutters, you can certainly use them, but they're not a necessity for making these savory-filled pillows. You'll be surprised at how easy to make these really are, and once you taste them, you'll be amazed they are actually Paleo friendly.

For the ravioli:
- 1 tablespoon olive oil
- 2 cups button mushrooms, finely chopped
- 1 pound baby spinach
- 1 recipe Paleo Pasta Dough

For the pesto:
- 2 cups packed basil leaves
- 2 cloves garlic
- Zest of 1 lemon
- 2 tablespoons pine nuts
- 4 tablespoons olive oil

Make the ravioli:

Heat a large skillet over medium heat. Add the olive oil and the mushrooms, and cook until lightly browned. Add the spinach and cook until wilted.

Divide the pasta into 2 pieces. Roll each piece out using a pasta maker until you have 2 sheets of pasta. Lay 1 sheet on a flat surface.

Add the ravioli filling to the dough in 1-teaspoon scoops about an inch apart, until you have no room left. Lay the other pasta sheet lightly on top.

Carefully cut around the balls of filling using a pizza cutter, and press the edges of each piece tightly shut.

Bring a large pot of water to a boil, add the ravioli, and reduce to a simmer. Cook for a few minutes, until the ravioli float to the top.

Make the pesto:

Combine all of the ingredients for the pesto in a food processor, and blend until you have a smooth sauce.

Once the ravioli are cooked, drain and serve topped with the pesto sauce.

Serves 4.

Pasta-Free Spaghetti and Meatballs

Pasta-free spaghetti? Yes, indeed! If you've never had spaghetti squash, you're in for a treat. With its pasta-like texture, it's the perfect substitute for the Paleo diet, and when paired with your favorite marinara sauce and meatballs, it will leave you so satisfied you'll never go back to carb-heavy, traditional pasta again!

- 2 spaghetti squash
- 4 cups prepared marinara sauce
- 2 tablespoons olive oil
- 1 small onion, chopped
- 2 cloves garlic, minced
- 1 tablespoon Italian seasoning
- ½ pound grass-fed beef, ground
- ½ pound free-range pork, ground
- ½ pound grass-fed veal, ground
- ½ cup almond flour
- 1 egg

Preheat oven to 375 degrees F.

Place the squash on a baking sheet, and bake for 30 minutes. Remove from oven and prick with a fork. Continue baking for 30 more minutes.

Pour the sauce in a medium saucepan, and simmer on low.

In a medium skillet, heat the olive oil over medium heat, and add the onion and garlic. Cook for 5 minutes and remove from heat.

In a large bowl, combine the Italian seasoning with all the ground meats, and mix gently with your hands. Add in the almond flour and egg, followed by the onion and garlic when cool.

Form the mixture into 2-inch meatballs, and lay on a parchment-lined baking sheet. Bake for 20 minutes. Remove from oven, and add the meatballs to the sauce to finish cooking.

When the squash are fully cooked, remove from oven, and carefully cut in half crosswise with a sharp knife.

Remove the seeds and pulp, and separate the "spaghetti" strands with a fork. Divide the squash between plates, and top with the hot sauce and meatballs.

Serves 4.

Shrimp and Garlic Fettuccini

This meal comes together extremely quickly, and it is a delicious meal for one of those extra-busy nights. The tender pasta and buttery garlic sauce are delectable accompaniments to the shrimp. The plain version of the Paleo Pasta Dough works perfectly well here, but any flavored version of your choice should be equally successful; roasted garlic or lemon pepper is especially nice. For an even speedier preparation, buy shrimp that are already peeled and deveined to save you the step of having to do this yourself.

- 1 recipe Paleo Pasta Dough, cut into fettuccini noodles
- 1 stick grass-fed butter
- 4 cloves garlic, minced
- 1 pound raw shrimp, peeled and deveined
- 1 large tomato, diced
- 1 bunch basil leaves, sliced, divided

Bring a large pot of salted water to a boil, and cook the noodles for about 20 seconds, being careful not to overcook. Drain and set aside.

Heat a large skillet over medium heat, and add the butter and garlic. Cook until the butter is melted and garlic is fragrant.

Add the shrimp and cook until just pink. Turn off heat and add the pasta. Toss until combined.

Stir in the tomatoes and half of the sliced basil.

To serve, divide the pasta and shrimp between 4 plates, and top with the remaining sliced basil to garnish.

Serves 4.

Pasta with Asparagus, Pancetta, and Eggs

This pasta dish is best served with a thinner noodle, so if you have a pasta machine, the Paleo Pasta Dough makes an excellent choice here. If you have a favorite Paleo-friendly dried pasta, that will work as well. The fried eggs add a nice, filling aspect to the meal, and you'll be surprised at how much flavor the slightly runny yolk adds to the hot pasta.

- 1 bunch asparagus, cut into bite-sized pieces
- 1 pound Paleo-friendly angel hair, or 1 recipe Paleo Pasta Dough, cut into thin noodles
- 2–3 slices high-quality pancetta, diced
- 4 large eggs
- 2 tablespoons grass-fed butter
- 1 bunch parsley, finely chopped

Bring a large pot of water to a boil, and add the asparagus. Cook for 2 minutes and remove with a slotted spoon. Add the pasta and cook according to the package directions. Drain and set aside.

Heat a large skillet over medium heat, and add the pancetta. Cook until crispy, and remove with a slotted spoon, leaving the fat in the pan.

Crack the eggs into the pan, cooking as many as will fit. Cook sunny-side up until the white is firm, but the yolk is still slightly runny. Remove from the pan, and add the butter.

When the butter is melted, add the pasta, cooked pancetta, and asparagus to the pan. Toss and add the parsley.

Dived the pasta onto plates, and top each serving with a fried egg.

Serves 4.

Pasta Primavera

It's no secret that vegetables are essential to the Paleo diet, and this easy pasta dish is loaded with them. This simple dish is amazing in the summertime when produce is abundant and fresh, but it's a treat any time of the year. Feel free to substitute whatever fresh veggies you have on hand: asparagus or green beans always make a pleasing addition. Use the Paleo Pasta Dough recipe for best results, or try one of the flavored versions—Fresh Herb or Roasted Garlic works especially well.

- ¼ cup olive oil
- 2 carrots, peeled and thinly sliced
- 1 zucchini, thinly sliced
- 1 onion, thinly sliced
- 1 red bell pepper, cut into strips
- 1 yellow bell pepper, cut into strips
- 1 tablespoon Italian seasoning
- 1 recipe Paleo Pasta Dough, cut into thin noodles
- 15–20 cherry tomatoes, halved
- Fresh basil, slivered, for garnish

In a large deep skillet, heat the olive oil over medium heat. Add the vegetables and stir to coat with the oil. Sauté until tender and stir in the Italian seasoning.

Bring a large pot of salted water to a boil, and add the noodles. Cook for 20–30 seconds, being careful not to overcook, and drain.

Add the cooked noodles to the sautéed vegetables, and turn off the heat. Add the cherry tomatoes and stir.

Divide between plates and top with the fresh basil to garnish.

Serves 4.

Spring Herb Pasta

This fresh and light pasta dish is a tempting early spring or summer meal. If you can enjoy it outdoors with friends, even better. The recipe calls for the Fresh Herb Pasta dough, but you can use the plain variety or any other recipe you like. This dish filled with bright green veggies is healthful, satisfying, and delicious, and perfect for company.

- 1 cup sliced green beans
- 1 cup pea pods
- 1 bunch asparagus, sliced
- 1 recipe Fresh Herb Pasta dough, cut into fettuccini noodles
- 2 tablespoons olive oil
- ¼ cup chopped green onions
- ¼ cup fresh herbs of your choice, chopped
- Juice of 1 lemon

Fill a large bowl with ice water.

Bring a pot of salted water to a boil, and add the vegetables. Cook for 2 minutes. Drain and plunge the vegetables into the ice-cold water. Allow to sit for a few minutes, then drain again.

Bring another salted pot of water to a boil, and add the noodles. Cook for 20 seconds, drain, and set aside.

Heat a large, deep skillet over medium heat. Add the olive oil and green onions, and cook for a minute until slightly soft. Add the herbs and stir.

Add the blanched veggies and cook for about 2 minutes, until heated through.

Add the cooked pasta and toss, then add the lemon juice and stir.

To serve, divide the pasta between 4 plates. Enjoy hot.

Serves 4.

Paleo Beef and Noodles

While the Paleo diet allows many of your favorite comfort foods, sometimes there is nothing better than a hot bowl of beef and noodles, especially on a cold winter night. This recipe, using the Paleo Pasta Dough provided earlier, allows you to enjoy your favorite comfort meal once again. For a richer, more authentic flavor, feel free to substitute a cup of red wine for a cup of beef broth, but if you're sticking strictly to your diet, you'll still find it very enjoyable without.

- 1 tablespoon olive oil
- 1 pound grass-fed beef stew meat, cubed
- 1 medium onion, chopped
- 2 cloves garlic, minced
- 5 cups beef broth, preferably homemade
- 2 teaspoons dried marjoram
- 1 recipe Paleo Pasta Dough, cut into thick 2-inch-long noodles

Heat the oil to medium-high heat in a large pot or Dutch oven. Add the beef and sear until browned on all sides, working in batches if necessary. Remove the meat from the pot and set aside.

Add the onion and garlic to the pot, and cook until soft. Add the meat back to the pot, followed by the broth and dried marjoram.

Bring to a boil and reduce heat. Simmer on low heat for about 2 hours, until the meat is tender.

When the meat is tender, add the noodles to the pot. Simmer for a few minutes, until noodles are tender. Serve hot.

Leftovers can be stored in the refrigerator for several days; simply reheat and enjoy again.

Serves 4.

Mixed Mushroom Pappardelle

Pappardelle is a long, fat noodle similar to fettuccini, but about three times its width. It pairs well with the richness and heartiness of the mushrooms in this dish. Buy whatever mushrooms you like here, but stick to fresh ones, as you'll get a much better flavor. To wash mushrooms, simply brush them off with a soft brush or paper towel, as rinsing them will prevent them from browning no matter how much you try to dry them.

- 1 recipe Paleo Pasta Dough, cut into long, wide noodles
- 2 tablespoons grass-fed butter
- 2 tablespoons olive oil
- 3 cups mixed mushrooms (such as cremini, oyster, or morel), sliced
- 1 clove garlic, minced
- Juice of 1 lemon, extra lemon wedges for garnish
- 1 bunch fresh parsley, chopped

Bring a large pot of salted water to a boil, and add the noodles. Cook for about 30 seconds and drain. Set aside.

Heat a large skillet over medium heat, and add the butter and olive oil. When the butter is melted, add the mushrooms. Cook until browned and soft, then add the garlic. Cook for 1 minute, and add the lemon juice.

Stir in the parsley, and add the cooked pasta. Toss until well combined.

To serve, divide between 4 plates. Serve hot with extra lemon wedges on the side and more fresh chopped parsley if desired.

Serves 4.

Fettuccini with Salmon and Lemon Dill Sauce

Tender chunks of salmon beautifully complement the buttery lemon dill sauce in this Paleo-friendly pasta dish. The entire meal comes together quickly, making an elegant weeknight dinner. If you're looking to impress guests, but don't want to disrupt your diet, this is a hit as well. You can use the Paleo Pasta Dough for this dish, but the version with spinach works nicely here as well. Make sure to buy wild salmon—not only is it the most flavorful, but it's also the only type approved by the Paleo diet.

- 1 recipe Paleo Pasta Dough, cut into fettuccini noodles
- 2 tablespoons butter
- 2 tablespoons olive oil
- 1 pound skinless wild salmon, cut into chunks
- 2 tablespoons fresh dill, chopped
- Juice and zest of 1 lemon
- 2 tablespoons capers

Bring a large pot of salted water to a boil. Cook the noodles for 20 seconds and drain. Set aside.

Heat a large skillet over medium-low heat, and add the butter and olive oil. When the butter is melted, add the salmon pieces. Allow the salmon to poach for a few minutes until cooked through.

Add the dill, lemon juice, and zest, and stir.

Add the cooked noodles, and toss well to combine. Stir in the capers.

Divide between plates and serve, topped with additional fresh chopped dill if desired.

Serves 4.

Sun-Dried Tomato and Arugula Linguine

Sun-dried tomatoes are full of flavor, and they complement the spicy arugula nicely in this simple pasta dish perfect for summer. The key to ensuring this dish has the right texture is topping the hot pasta with the arugula at the table and stirring it gently. The arugula gets slightly wilted, but not slimy and overcooked. It's a delicate balance of flavors that makes a refined weeknight meal. If you're looking for something a little more filling, add some cooked shrimp or chicken.

- 1 recipe Paleo Pasta Dough, cut into linguine noodles
- 4 tablespoons olive oil
- 4 cloves garlic, minced
- ½ cup sun-dried tomatoes, sliced
- 4 cups fresh arugula leaves, chopped

Bring a large pot of salted water to a boil, and cook the noodles for about 15 seconds, being careful not to overcook. Drain and set aside.

Heat a large skillet over medium heat, and add the olive oil and garlic. Cook until garlic is fragrant, about 1 minute.

Add the sun-dried tomatoes. Turn off heat and add the pasta. Toss until combined.

To serve, divide the pasta between plates, and top each plate with 1 cup of the arugula leaves. Stir slightly just before eating.

Serves 4.

Roasted Root Vegetable Pappardelle

Tender, sweet root vegetables paired with a delicious Paleo pasta make a healthful meal that is wonderfully hearty in the winter months. Feel free to use whatever veggies you happen to have on hand, although the variety here is particularly successful. This dish makes excellent use of leftover vegetables from a previous meal; simply reheat and toss with the cooked pasta.

- 1 medium turnip, peeled and cut into bite-sized pieces
- 1 medium parsnip, peeled and cut into bite-sized pieces
- 1 medium beet, peeled and cut into bite-sized pieces
- 1 medium sweet potato, peeled and cut into bite-sized pieces
- 2 tablespoons olive oil
- 1 teaspoon dried thyme
- 1 recipe Paleo Pasta Dough, cut into long, wide noodles
- ¼ cup walnuts, chopped and toasted

Preheat oven to 400 degrees F.

Toss the vegetables with the olive oil and thyme, and lay on a parchment-lined sheet pan in a single layer.

Roast for 45–50 minutes, until the vegetables are lightly browned and tender.

Bring a large pot of salted water to a boil, and add the noodles. Cook for 30 seconds and drain.

Toss the hot cooked noodles with the roasted vegetables and the toasted walnuts.

Serve immediately.

Serves 4.

PALEO BAKED PASTAS

Paleo Lasagna

Even though there's no cheese in this classic Italian casserole, it is still full of flavor—a Paleo nut "cheese" adds a lovely taste and familiar creaminess. It's also remarkably easy to prepare using fresh pasta that doesn't need to be boiled before baking. If you don't have a pasta maker, roll the pasta as thin as you possibly can between two sheets of parchment paper.

- 1 pound grass-fed beef, ground
- 1 medium onion, chopped
- 2 cups button mushrooms, sliced
- 6 cups prepared marinara sauce
- 1 cup raw walnuts
- ½ cup raw pumpkin seeds
- ½ cup raw pecans
- ½ cup unsweetened almond milk
- ¼ teaspoon ground nutmeg
- 1 recipe Paleo Pasta Dough, rolled through a pasta maker in thin sheets

Preheat oven to 350 degrees F.

Heat a medium saucepan over medium-high heat and add the ground beef. Break it up as it cooks, and add the onion and mushrooms.

Sauté onion until translucent and mushrooms are slightly browned. Pour in the marinara sauce, and turn the heat down to medium-low to simmer.

While the sauce simmers, make the "cheese" sauce by combining the walnuts, pumpkin seeds, and pecans in a food processor with the almond milk and nutmeg. Blend until smooth, adding more almond milk if necessary. It should become the consistency of ricotta cheese.

Once your "cheese" is done, assemble the lasagna by layering the ingredients in a 9 x 13–inch casserole dish in the following order: pasta, sauce, "cheese." Keep layering until you have used these up, and the top is covered with sauce.

Bake the lasagna uncovered for about 1 hour, until the top becomes browned and bubbly. Allow the lasagna to rest for 10 minutes before slicing and serving.

Leftovers can be stored in the refrigerator for several days.

Serves 6 to 8.

Paleo Baked Macaroni

There are many brands of gluten-free pasta compatible with the Paleo diet; just remember that some may contain corn or rice. Check labels to find a brand suitable to you, and eat it sparingly when you have a craving for pasta. This baked macaroni dish comes together extremely easily, and you'll get a rich, creamy flavor from the "cheese" sauce mixed through it.

- 1 pound Paleo-friendly dried macaroni
- 1 cup raw walnuts
- ½ cup raw pumpkin seeds
- ½ cup raw pecans
- 1 cup unsweetened almond milk
- ¼ teaspoon ground nutmeg
- 4 cups prepared marinara sauce

Preheat oven to 350 degrees F.

Cook the pasta according to the package directions. Drain and set aside.

Make the "cheese" sauce by combining the walnuts, pumpkin seeds, and pecans in a food processor with the almond milk and nutmeg. Blend until smooth, adding more almond milk if necessary. It should become the consistency of a thick cream sauce.

Combine the pasta with the "cheese" sauce and the marinara sauce. Pour into a 9 x 13–inch casserole dish, and cover with foil.

Bake for 45 minutes. Remove from oven and allow to sit for 5 minutes before serving.

Store leftovers in the refrigerator for up to 3 days.

Serves 6 to 8.

Eggplant "Lasagna"

This casserole dish will remind you of lasagna in the way it is prepared and baked, but the secret of its success is the tender eggplant that replaces the starchy noodles. A mandolin works best here for slicing the eggplant as thin as possible, but a sharp knife will do the job if you take your time. Slice the eggplant lengthwise for a more traditional lasagna shape, but if you think it's easier to slice it into rounds, that will work as well. This makes excellent leftovers, so don't be afraid to make this recipe even if you're cooking for only two.

- 1 pound grass-fed beef, ground
- 1 medium onion, chopped
- 2 cups button mushrooms, sliced
- 6 cups prepared marinara sauce
- 1 cup raw walnuts
- ½ cup raw pumpkin seeds
- ½ cup raw pecans
- ½ cup unsweetened almond milk
- ¼ teaspoon ground nutmeg
- 4 cups frozen spinach, thawed and chopped
- 1 large eggplant

Preheat oven to 350 degrees F.

Heat a medium saucepan over medium-high heat and add the ground beef. Break it up as it cooks, and add the onion and mushrooms.

Sauté onion until translucent and the mushrooms are slightly browned. Pour in the marinara sauce, and turn the heat down from medium-high to simmer.

While the sauce simmers, make the "cheese" sauce by combining the walnuts, pumpkin seeds, and pecans in a food processor with the almond milk and nutmeg. Blend until smooth, adding more almond milk if necessary. It should become the consistency of ricotta cheese. Add the spinach to this mixture, and stir until well combined.

Using a mandolin or sharp knife, slice the eggplant lengthwise in about ¼-inch-thick slices.

Once your cheese is done, make the lasagna by layering the ingredients in a 9 x 13–inch casserole dish in the following order: eggplant, sauce, "cheese." Keep layering until you have used these up, and the top is covered with sauce.

Bake the lasagna uncovered for about 1 hour, until the top becomes browned and bubbly. Allow the lasagna to rest for 10 minutes before slicing and serving.

Leftovers can be stored in the refrigerator for several days.

Serves 6 to 8.

Baked Penne with Tuna

High-quality tuna and tender, Paleo-friendly pasta make a hearty meal that's both comforting and filling on a cold night. This baked dish is best prepared with a penne or fusilli-type pasta; for suggested brands, check the Resources section in this book. Use high-quality tuna packed in oil instead of the water-packed cans for a richer flavor.

- 1 pound Paleo-friendly pasta, such as penne or fusilli
- 12 ounces high-quality flaked tuna, drained
- 3 cups diced tomatoes
- 2 tablespoons olive oil
- 1 cup unsweetened almond milk
- 1 cup raw walnuts
- ½ cup raw pecans
- ½ cup raw pumpkin seeds
- ¼ teaspoon ground nutmeg
- Fresh chopped parsley, for garnish

Preheat oven to 350 degrees F.

Cook the pasta according to the directions on the package; drain and set aside.

In a large bowl, combine the tuna with the tomatoes and olive oil. Set aside.

Put the almond milk, nuts, seeds, and nutmeg in a food processor, and process until you have a smooth sauce—it should resemble a thick cream sauce. Pour this over the tomatoes and tuna, and stir to combine.

Add the pasta and stir. Transfer everything to a 9 x 13–inch casserole dish, and cover with foil.

Bake for 45 minutes. Remove from oven and allow to sit for 5 minutes before serving.

Serve topped with the chopped parsley.

Serves 6 to 8.

Penne Pasta Bake

Unlike many baked pasta dishes, this one is on the lighter side but still full of flavor. The sauce is creamy and buttery, and it pairs nicely with the zucchini and Paleo-friendly pasta. Be careful not to overcook the pasta, or you'll end up with a casserole that's mushy instead of tender and slightly firm.

- 1 pound Paleo-friendly penne pasta
- 2 tablespoons olive oil
- 1 medium zucchini, sliced into ½-inch rounds
- 1 clove garlic, minced
- 2 tablespoons grass-fed butter
- 4 tablespoons almond flour
- 2 cups unsweetened almond milk
- ¼ teaspoon ground nutmeg
- 1 teaspoon Dijon mustard

Preheat oven to 350 degrees F.

Cook the pasta according to the package directions, making sure you don't overcook it. Drain and set aside.

In a medium saucepan, heat the olive oil to medium-high heat and add the zucchini. Cook until soft, about 2 minutes. Add the garlic and cook for 1 more minute.

Add the butter and stir. When the butter is melted, add the almond flour and stir for 1 minute. Add the almond milk, nutmeg, and mustard, and stir until creamy.

Put the cooked pasta in a 9 x 13–inch casserole dish, and pour the sauce over the top, making sure all of the pasta is covered.

Cover the dish with foil, and bake for 30 minutes. Remove from oven and let sit for 5 minutes. Serve hot.

Store leftovers in the fridge for up to 3 days.

Serves 6 to 8.

Spicy Sausage Bake

This hearty pasta dish needs a noodle that is hearty enough to stand up to the spicy sauce and Italian sausage. A good Paleo-friendly rigatoni is best, but a penne will do. Make sure to buy the highest quality sausage you can find and remove the casings if necessary. This is an easy-to-assemble dish you can bring to a potluck or other gathering—and it's unlikely anyone will guess it's Paleo approved. It can also be prepared in advance, then baked whenever you need it, making a great meal for busy weeknights.

- 1 pound high-quality, spicy Italian sausage, casings removed
- 2 tablespoons fresh parsley, chopped
- 1 teaspoon crushed red pepper flakes
- 3 cups prepared marinara sauce
- 1 pound Paleo-friendly pasta, such as rigatoni or penne

Preheat oven to 350 degrees F.

Heat a Dutch oven or saucepot over medium heat. Add the sausage and cook until browned, crumbling as you go. Stir in the parsley and red pepper flakes, and continue cooking until sausage is well browned.

Pour the marinara sauce over the sausage, and bring to a simmer.

Meanwhile, cook the pasta according to the package directions, making sure not to overcook. Drain and add to the marinara sauce.

Transfer the sauce-coated pasta to a 9 x 13–inch casserole dish, and cover with foil.

Bake for 30 minutes, and remove from oven. Allow to sit for 5 minutes before serving.

Store leftovers in the refrigerator for up to 3 days.

Serves 6 to 8.

Chicken and Broccoli Penne

Tender chunks of chicken and broccoli pair beautifully with the creamy "cheese" sauce in this pasta dish. While there are many gluten-free pastas on the market, not all are Paleo friendly, so take a look at the labels to decide which ones best fit your lifestyle. Check the Resources section in this book for various brands and what they have to offer.

- 1 pound Paleo-friendly penne pasta
- 2 tablespoons butter
- 2 tablespoons olive oil
- 1 pound free-range chicken breasts, cut into bite-sized pieces
- 2 cups broccoli florets, cut into small pieces
- 1 cup unsweetened almond milk
- 1 cup raw walnuts
- ½ cup raw pecans
- ½ cup raw pumpkin seeds
- ¼ teaspoon ground nutmeg

Preheat oven to 350 degrees F.

Cook the pasta according to the package directions. Drain and set aside.

Heat the butter and olive oil in a deep skillet to medium heat. Add the chicken and cook until browned. Add the broccoli and toss. Cook for 3 minutes. Turn off heat.

Combine the almond milk with the nuts, seeds, and nutmeg in a food processor, and puree until you have a smooth sauce. Add this to the chicken and broccoli mixture and stir well.

Transfer the cooked pasta to a 9 x 13–inch casserole dish, and pour the chicken and broccoli mixture over the top. Stir to mix well.

Cover with foil and bake for 45 minutes. Remove from the oven, and allow to sit for 10 minutes before serving.

Store leftovers in the refrigerator for up to 3 days.

Serves 6 to 8.

SECTION TWO

The Basics of the Paleo Diet

WHAT IS THE PALEO DIET?

Whether modern health-care professionals want to admit it or not, the Paleo diet closely mirrors what most of them tell their patients: eat more fruits, vegetables, and lean meats, and stay away from processed garbage. The diet, also known as the Stone Age diet, the caveman diet, and the hunter-gatherer diet, has gained a significant following in recent years, and there's some pretty good research to support the switch.

How Did the Paleo Diet Start?

Back in the 1970s a gastroenterologist by the name of Walter L. Voegtlin observed that digestive diseases such as colitis, Crohn's disease, and irritable bowel syndrome were much more prevalent in people who followed a modern Western diet than they were in people's ancestors, whose diet consisted largely of vegetables, fruits, nuts, and lean meats. He began treating patients with these disorders by recommending diets low in carbohydrates and high in animal fats.

Unfortunately, the medical world simply wasn't ready to give up the idea that a low-fat, low-calorie diet was the healthiest way to eat, so Dr. Voegtlin's observations and research went largely unnoticed, and the Paleo diet was shoved to the back of the drawer.

Finally—The Stone Age Is Cool Again!

Fast-forward a decade to a point when medical researchers had gained considerably more insight into how the human body actually works. Melvin Konner, S. Boyd Eaton, and Marjorie Shostak of Emory University published a book called *The Paleolithic Prescription: A Program of Diet and Exercise and a Design for Living,* then followed it up with a second book, *The Stone-Age Health Programme: Diet and Exercise as Nature Intended.* The first book became the foundation for most of the modern versions of the Paleo diet, and the second backed it up with more research.

The main difference was that instead of eliminating any foods that people's ancestors wouldn't have had access to as Dr. Voegtlin did originally, Konner, Eaton, and Shostak encouraged eating foods that were nutritionally and proportionally similar to a traditional caveman diet. Because it was more realistic, the diet caught on like wildfire, and the research in favor of it continues to grow.

What Are the Rules?

Paleo is one of the easiest diets on the planet to follow: just remember to keep it real. If it's processed, artificial, or otherwise not directly from the earth, don't eat it. It's that simple. Here's a list of the delicious, healthful foods that the Paleo diet encourages:

- Eggs
- Healthful oils—olive and coconut are best; canola oil is under debate right now, too
- Lean animal proteins
- Nuts and seeds (note, however, that peanuts are NOT nuts)
- Organic fruits
- Organic vegetables
- Seafood, especially cold-water fish such as salmon and tuna in order to get the most omega-3 fatty acids

Sounds kind of familiar, doesn't it? That's because it's probably what your doctor encouraged you to eat more of the last time that you went to see him or her! Now let's take a look at some foods that are off the table if you're going to eat Stone Age style:

- Alcohol
- Artificial foods, such as preservatives and zero-calorie sweeteners
- Cereal grains, such as wheat, barley, hops, corn, oats, rye, and rice
- Dairy (though some followers allow dairy for the health benefits)
- Legumes (including peanuts)
- Processed foods, such as wheat flour and sugar
- Processed meats, such as bacon, deli meats, sausage, and canned meats
- Starchy vegetables (though these are currently under debate)

Frequently Asked Questions

Now that you have a general idea of what you can and can't eat, you may still have a few questions, so here's a list of those most frequently asked.

Q. Why do I have to quit drinking?

A. Beer is basically liquid grain, and it's packed with empty calories. Many types of alcoholic products contain gluten, which is discussed in detail in Chapter 6. Mixed drinks and wine are often loaded with sugar. If you absolutely can't go without that Friday-night cocktail, shoot for red wine, tequila, potato vodka, or white rum—and be careful what you mix it with.

Q. Why are legumes forbidden? They're natural foods and great sources of protein.

A. Most legumes, in their raw state, are toxic. They contain lectins—proteins that bind carbohydrates and have been shown to cause such autoimmune diseases as lupus and rheumatoid arthritis. The phytates in many legumes inhibit your absorption of critical minerals, and the protease inhibitors interfere with how your body breaks down protein.

Q. Why no dairy?

A. This one's under debate and there are many Paleo followers who still incorporate dairy regularly into their diets. The main reason that dairy is generally forbidden is that humans are the only animals who drink milk as adults, and many food allergies and digestive disorders are lactose related. There's a much more scientific answer for this question, but it boils down to believing or not believing that milk is bad for you.

Q. How will I lose weight eating fat?

A. This is a question that most people have initially because you're programmed to believe that red meat is bad for your heart. The fact is lean, organic, free-range meat is an excellent source of protein and many other vitamins and minerals. You're not going to be living on it alone; you're going to be incorporating it into a healthful diet.

Q. Peanuts are nuts and corn is a vegetable, so why are they off-limits?

A. *Au contraire.* Peanuts are legumes and corn is a grain. Be careful that you know what food groups everything you eat falls into or you may sabotage your efforts to be healthier.

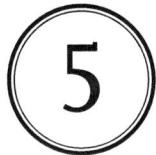

THE BENEFITS OF PALEO

Many people turn to the Paleo diet because of the weight-loss benefits, but that's not where the idea originated. If you remember, the diet was created by a gastroenterologist to help his patients with various gastric disorders. Of course, weight loss is a wonderful side effect that has its own set of healthful benefits.

When you add in the myriad other perks, going caveman is almost a no-brainer. Let's take a quick peek at some of the biggest health benefits of following a Paleo diet.

Weight Loss

Since this is one of the primary reasons that many people decide to switch to a Paleo diet, this is a good place to start. Because you're eliminating empty carbs and adding in lots of healthful plant fiber and lean protein, losing weight will be much easier. A few other factors that contribute to healthful weight loss include:

- Plant fiber takes longer to digest, so you feel full longer.
- Lean proteins help keep your energy levels steady while you build muscle.

- Omega-3s help boost your metabolism and reduce body fat.
- You'll be eating a greater volume of food but taking in fewer calories.

The bottom line is that you'll be consuming foods that help your body function the way that it's supposed to, and one of the natural side effects of that is weight loss.

Healthy Digestive System

Remember that this was the original reason for the diet to be utilized. The theory is that people's bodies aren't adapted to eating grains, dairy, and other foods that are forbidden by the Paleo diet, and so they cause digestive upset, inflammation, and discomfort. Also, your digestive tract needs fiber to help it sweep food through your system or else it builds up and causes problems. Just some of the conditions that may be improved by going caveman include:

- Colitis
- Constipation
- Gas
- Heartburn
- Irritable bowel syndrome

Many people who begin the Paleo diet for other reasons, such as weight loss or heart health, report improved digestive health. Yet another reason that this incredible diet is worth your time!

Type 2 Diabetes Prevention

In the United States and other cultures that have adopted a Western diet, type 2 diabetes has reached disastrous proportions. Historically an adult disease, children are developing this debilitating illness at an alarming rate, and there's no sign of this trend changing. One of the main culprits is excess consumption of processed sugars and flours.

By simply eliminating these calorie-laden, nutritionless foods from your diet, you can literally save your own life. The Paleo diet helps you avoid type 2 diabetes as well as metabolic syndrome, a precursor to many different diseases, for the following reasons:

- Omega-3s help reduce belly fat, an indicator of diabetes and metabolic syndrome.
- Lean proteins and plant fiber help increase insulin resistance so that your sugar levels don't spike.
- The vitamin C that's so readily available in citrus fruits and colorful veggies helps reduce belly fat.
- Lean protein takes longer to metabolize so you avoid energy highs and lows.

Immune Health

When you eat foods that your body isn't adapted to, such as processed grains, legumes, and dairy products, your body produces an allergic response in the form of inflammation, even if you don't experience any obvious outward symptoms. You may notice dark circles under your eyes as well as a feeling of general lethargy. You may attribute these symptoms to stress or exhaustion, but they're actually signs of a chronic allergy.

Inflammation in your body is a bad thing if it's occurring chronically, and it has been causally linked to such autoimmune disorders as:

- Fibromyalgia
- Lupus
- Multiple sclerosis
- Rheumatoid arthritis
- Several different types of cancer

The sad part here is that you don't even realize what you're doing to your body because there are often no symptoms until you have developed the disease. Switching to the Paleo diet may help reduce or eliminate your risk of many debilitating illnesses.

Cardiovascular Health

For most of your life, you've probably been told how horrible red meat and other animal proteins are for your heart, but recent research indicates that this is simply not true. Remember that there's a huge difference in scarfing down a fatty hamburger or sausage and enjoying a lean, organic, grass-fed steak. The burger and sausage are full of saturated fats and, most likely, hormones and additives.

On the other hand, steak is a lean, nutritious protein that delivers essential vitamins and minerals with very little bad fat and no empty calories, preservatives, or hormones. When you throw omega-3s and LDL-lowering healthful fats into the mix, you've got a heart-healthful meal that's good for anybody.

A Few Final Words on Health

The health benefits of giving up processed flour, refined sugar, and foods that cause inflammatory responses could fill an entire doctoral thesis, and the advantages to eliminating hormones and artificial additives from foods could fill another one. This chapter didn't even touch on how a Paleo diet can help with allergies, cancer, brain health, joint health, or celiac disease, but some of these will be covered in the discussion of the health risks of gluten in the next chapter. Suffice to say, the benefits of going Paleo far outweigh the relatively minor inconvenience of giving up a few foods.

6

THE TROUBLE WITH GLUTEN

Of the many health benefits of switching to a Paleo diet, one of the main benefits is that foods allowed on the diet don't have gluten in them. For millions of people worldwide, eating caveman-style is a relatively simple way to avoid digestive upset and even cancers that are caused by an allergy to gluten.

What Is Gluten?

Latin for "glue," gluten is a protein found in wheat and grains that gives the ground flours elasticity and helps them to rise. It's also the binding component that gives bread its chewy texture and keeps it from crumbling apart after baking. Because gluten is insoluble in water, it can be removed from flour, but typically when you do that, you lose all of the good properties that make breads and cakes what they are.

Without gluten, your baked goods won't rise and they'll have a grainy, crumbly texture. They won't taste anything like their gluten-laden cousins, and you probably won't want to eat more after the first bite. Because of an increasing demand for gluten-free products, food corporations have dedicated a tremendous amount of time and money into creating tasty, effective gluten-free products. Unfortunately, most commercially prepared gluten-free recipe mixes still fall short.

Is the Paleo Diet Gluten-Free?

Because gluten naturally occurs in wheat and grains, the Paleo diet is completely gluten-free. All grain products are strictly forbidden. Remember, the original creator of the diet was a gastroenterologist developing a plan that would help his patients with gastric disorders. Gluten intolerance is one of the most prevalent causes of gastrointestinal distress in Western civilization.

What Is Gluten Intolerance?

Gluten intolerance, or celiac disease in its advanced stage, is a condition that damages the small intestine, and it's triggered by eating foods that have gluten in them. Some of these foods include:

- Bread
- Cookies
- Just about any baked goods
- Most flours, including white and wheat flours
- Pasta
- Pizza dough

Gluten triggers an immune response in the small intestine that causes damage to its inside. This can lead to an inability to absorb vital nutrients. Other illnesses associated with this disease include lactose intolerance, bone loss, several types of cancer, neurological complications, and malnutrition. Diseases notwithstanding, just the symptoms of gluten intolerance can disrupt daily life. They include:

- Depression
- Fatigue
- Joint pain
- Neuropathy

- Osteoporosis
- Rashes
- Severe diarrhea
- Stomach cramps

These are only a few of the symptoms that a person with gluten intolerance can suffer from, and since all foods that contain gluten are forbidden on the Paleo diet, you can see what the appeal is.

The Harmful Effects of Gluten

Gluten doesn't just harm people with fully developed celiac disease. It's actually harmful to us all. Long-term studies indicate that people who have even a mild sensitivity to gluten exhibit a significantly higher risk of death than people who do not. The worst part is that 99 percent of people with gluten sensitivity don't even know they have it. They attribute their symptoms to other conditions, such as stress or fatigue.

Absorption Malfunction

One of the attributes that many obese or overweight people share is the fact that they can still feel hungry after eating a full meal. This feeling of hunger is because gluten sensitivity is preventing your body from absorbing vital nutrients.

Food Addiction

There are chemicals called exorphins in some foods that cause you to crave food even when you're not hungry. Food addiction is a serious issue and doesn't necessarily denote a lack of willpower; these exorphins are actually a drug-like chemical released in your brain that creates an irresistible desire for more food. Gluten contains as many as fifteen different exorphins.

Though food companies have created gluten-free foods, they often replace the gluten with flavor-enhancers, such as sodium and sugar, which can still seriously sabotage your dieting and fitness efforts. Another advantage to the Paleo diet is that by following it, you're not only eliminating gluten, you're also avoiding the pitfalls of commercially prepared foods that continue to make you sick.

Other Conditions Related to Gluten

There are numerous other conditions related to gluten sensitivity, and many professionals postulate that this is simply because people's bodies aren't adapted to eating grains so they are treated as allergens. Other symptoms or disorders linked to eating gluten include:

- Anxiety
- Autism
- Dementia
- Migraines
- Mouth sores
- Schizophrenia
- Seizures

These aren't just minor aches and pains, though gluten sensitivity can cause those, too. These are major diseases and conditions that can ruin your life. It's no wonder that people who know that they suffer from gluten intolerance consider the Paleo diet.

Health Benefits of Going Gluten-Free

Obviously, there are countless benefits of giving up gluten, but here are a few that may be of particular interest to you:

- Decreased chance of several types of cancer

- Healthy, painless digestion
- Healthy skin
- Improved brain function
- Improved mood
- Reduced appetite
- Weight loss (or gain, if you're underweight because of malnutrition)

With the obvious advantages of giving up grains, it's difficult to understand exactly why people would hesitate. It's just a matter of making some adjustments to your diet, and now that understanding about both food and health is increasing, there are some great alternatives out there that will help you get rid of your addiction to grains!

$$\bigg(7\bigg)$$

PALEO FOOD GUIDE

S hopping for foods that are Paleo friendly can be a daunting task when you're first starting out. What's allowed and what's not? What are all of those mystery ingredients that are listed in foods? For the most part, stocking your fridge and pantry is fairly simple, but there are going to be times when you don't want to eat just steak and broccoli, and there will be other times when you need something fast and simple. Don't worry: you'll get the hang of it.

There are a few different versions of the Paleo diet, but this discussion will focus on the modern middle road so that it's easier for you to make the transition to your new, healthier lifestyle. Throughout the following paragraphs, you'll learn what foods are OK and where you can find them. You'll also learn some alternate ingredients for baking muffins and other goodies that won't get you kicked out of the cave!

Paleo Pantry and Kitchen Tips

The first bit of good news is that you're not going to be counting calories. Instead, you're going to try to keep your portions in line with what your ancestors most likely ate. A diet that consists of 50 to 60 percent protein,

30 to 45 percent healthful carbs, and 5 to 10 percent healthful vegetable fats, such as olive oil, avocados, nuts, and seeds, is the general goal.

Basically, when you're stacking your plate, put your protein on one side and your fruits and veggies on the other. Snacks can be whatever you want, but veggies and nuts are great choices. Be careful with nuts and fruits; though they're good for you, they're high in calories and can sabotage your weight-loss efforts if you're not careful.

If Possible, Go Raw

Many fruits and vegetables lose nutritional value when you cook them, so when possible, eat them raw. You'll also eat less because you'll be chewing more. If you opt to cook your veggies, steam them lightly so they maintain their bright colors. A key clue that you've cooked your greens to death is that they've lost that pretty vibrant green hue and turned an olive color. Try to avoid that.

Steaming, baking, grilling, and broiling are all great methods of cooking and require little added fat to prevent sticking. It should go without saying that the fryer can be retired to the garage to be sold at your next rummage sale.

Cooking on the Fly

Meals away from home can be a real challenge when you're first starting out. Restaurants are filled with tempting burgers and fries, and you have no idea what's in the salad dressings. If you must eat out, order a plain garden salad with oil and vinegar. You could also request a steak or chicken breast to go on top, but make sure that they either grill it dry or use olive oil.

Opt not to eat out in the beginning. Instead, make an amazing soup at home for dinner with enough leftover that you aren't tempted to go out for a quick fix. That way, you know what's in your food and you know that it's going to be delicious!

Plan Ahead

If you know in advance what you're going to eat for lunch or for dinner, you're not going to be as likely to cheat with something quick from the vending machine. Take snacks to work with you so that the box of doughnuts isn't so tempting.

Meats and Proteins

Your meats need to come from grass-fed, organic livestock, free-range poultry, or wild-caught fish and seafood. Wild game is great, too, if you're so inclined. Actually, meats such as venison are extremely low in bad fats and high in good fats and lean protein, so feel free to partake!

Fruits and Vegetables

If at all possible, shop at your local farmers' market for fresh organic fruits and veggies. Since the Paleo diet is dependent upon your creativity to complete a hot, fresh, delicious meal without the aid of flours, fats, and no-no's, you're going to have to learn a number of ways to prepare dishes. Plus, if you're offering a wide variety of foods that your family knows and loves, you won't be under so much pressure to create a single main dish that everybody will eat and enjoy.

Tomatoes are a great addition to any salad and make a flavorful base for soups and sauces. They're packed with nutrients and have so many uses that you should always have some on hand. Other staples should include carrots, peppers, cauliflower, and celery.

For fruits, opt for ones that are high in nutrients and relatively low in sugar, such as stone fruits and berries. Berries are also fabulous sources of antioxidants, phytonutrients, and vitamins. Apples are an easy grab-and-go food, as are peaches, oranges, and bananas. The dark tip of the banana that you usually pick off is rich in vitamin K, so eat it!

Oils and Fats

Oils high in saturated fats, such as corn oil and vegetable oil, are out. Opt instead for oils that are high in omega-3s, such as olive oil, avocado oil, coconut oil, and possibly canola oil. The latter is currently a point of contention among long-term Paleo followers, but there's a compelling argument to include it.

Seasonings

Your success with making the transition to the caveman way of eating is largely dependent on how flavorful your food is. As a result, you're going to need to incorporate various herbs and spices to make your dishes delicious. Here are a few that you should always have on hand:

- Allspice
- Black pepper
- Basil
- Cayenne pepper
- Cinnamon
- Cloves
- Crushed red pepper
- Curry powder
- Dry mustard
- Garlic—fresh and powdered
- Mustard seed
- Oregano
- Paprika

- Parsley
- Rosemary
- Thyme

Snacks

Finally, you'll probably want to keep some snacks on hand. Now, that does NOT mean cupcakes, potato chips, or crackers. However, there are still many options, such as certain beef jerky (or even better, make your own!), dried fruits, nuts, and seeds. They're satisfying and add nutrients to your diet instead of unhealthful fats.

Paleo Shopping Tips

Going to the grocery store is going to be a bit of a challenge at first, just as it is anytime that you make changes to your diet. Especially if you're accustomed to eating a large amount of refined flour and sugar and aren't yet over your sugar addiction, it's not going to be easy. Here are a few tips to help you along your way.

- Shop for your produce at the local farmers' market if possible.
- When at the grocery store, shop around the perimeter of the store. That's where most stores keep all of their meats and produce, and 99 percent of your food is going to come from those departments. If you need to get something from an aisle, go straight in, get it, and get back to the perimeter before those cookies catch your eye!
- Make a list and stick to it.
- If you do choose to eat canned fruits and veggies, make sure that you read the label so that you're not getting hidden sodium and preservatives.
- Buy meat in bulk when you catch a sale.
- Don't shop hungry! Have a low-fat, high-protein snack before you go so that you aren't tempted while you're there.

CONCLUSION

Whatever your personal reasons behind your decision to pursue the Paleo lifestyle, you made the right choice, even though making the switch from a Western diet may seem a bit tough at the start. Many of the foods and ingredients you've likely considered cooking, as well as the dietary staples you've relied on all your life, are no longer permitted. But if you're fairly creative and willing to try new things, you're going to discover some really fantastic alternatives.

Finding a replacement for pasta is a challenge because nothing is going to taste exactly like noodles made from gluten-laden wheat. The trick to creating dishes you really enjoy is to give up the notion of locating something that tastes identical to traditional pasta, and focus instead on making wonderful-tasting Paleo pastas reminiscent of those unhealthful pre-Paleo meals. After all, just because a pear doesn't taste like an apple doesn't mean it's not fruity and fabulous in its own right.

If you approach these recipes for gluten-free Paleo pastas from that perspective, you'll find yourself much happier than if you expect them to taste exactly like old-school noodles. As you try these dishes, you're probably going to be tasting new foods and experiencing textures that may seem unfamiliar, but the flavor combinations are out of this world if you simply give them a chance.

While each Paleo pasta recipe presented here is amazing in its original state, you should use this cookbook as a jumping-off point for your own new culinary experiences. First try the dishes exactly as the recipes are written; then as you become more comfortable working with the ingredients, begin to experiment with them. Make a dish once with dried spices, then with fresh ones to see how this affects the flavor. Or if you don't like mushrooms, try replacing them with olives or onions, or any other ingredient you absolutely love.

You're going to find that the more you experiment, the more you'll love these new, healthful dishes you create. So take these recipes, and make them your own. From the Paleo test kitchen to yours, best wishes for happy, healthful eating!

RESOURCES

Ingredients

Almond milk: Widely available in your grocer's dairy case, almond milk is simply ground almonds and filtered water. Unless stated otherwise, most brands contain added sweeteners, so be sure to buy unsweetened varieties. This is especially important when making savory pasta sauces, as the added sugars will ruin your dish.

Almond flour: Used as a substitute for wheat flour to thicken up sauces, almond flour is simply blanched almonds that are finely ground.

Arrowroot starch: A gluten-free powder and thickener, arrowroot starch is used in the pasta dough recipes in this book. It may be labeled arrow-root powder, starch, or flour—all are the same.

Coconut flour: Dried coconut that is ground into flour, coconut flour is used for the pasta recipes in this book. You should not substitute almond flour for coconut flour or vice versa, unless otherwise specified.

Flaxseed: Ground flax is the resulting powder when flaxseeds are finely ground, and it is the base of the homemade pasta recipes in this book. Regular flax is brown in color, but you can buy golden flaxseed if you would like your pasta to be lighter in color. The nutrition content and flavor of both is about the same.

Raw nuts: When blended with liquid such as almond milk or water, raw nuts produce a cheese-like sauce that makes a nice ricotta substitute. Make sure to buy only raw nuts for this purpose, as roasted nuts will give you a different texture and flavor.

Gluten-Free Paleo-Friendly Pasta

Ancient Harvest is a company that makes gluten-free pastas and other products suitable for a gluten-free diet. While their pastas are gluten-free, they do contain corn flour, so they are not ideal for the strictest of Paleo diets. For more information, visit www.quinoa.net.

Cappello's is a Colorado-based company that specializes in gluten- and grain-free pastas. For more information, go to www.cappellosglutenfree.com.

Miracle Noodle makes gluten- and grain-free noodles in all shapes and sizes suitable for a Paleo diet. For more information or to purchase some, go to www.miraclenoodle.com.

Paleo Pasta is a brand of gluten-free pasta made from fruits, vegetables, nuts, and other Paleo-friendly ingredients. You can find more information about their products at www.paleopasta.com.

Sources

Amazon is a Web marketplace where you can find Paleo-friendly products of all types. Most of the items you need for this book can be found at www.amazon.com and sometimes for lower prices than you'll find locally.

Bob's Red Mill is an all-natural brand of gluten-free flours, shredded coconut, and other dried or powdered ingredients. You can find many of their products in your local grocery store's baking aisle, or at www.bobsredmill.com.

Celtic Sea Salt is a maker of authentic, unprocessed sea salt, which will enhance the flavors of your baked goods. Go to www.celticseasalt.com for more information on their products, as well as where they can be purchased.

Spectrum Naturals is a brand of all-natural, organic oils available at grocers nationwide. Go to www.spectrumorganics.com for more information on their coconut oil, palm shortening, and other high-quality products.

Whole Foods Market is the world's largest natural food store with a variety of gluten-free and Paleo-friendly products. For locations, go to www.wholefoodsmarket.com.

CPSIA information can be obtained at www.ICGtesting.com
Printed in the USA
LVOW06s1817290813

350196LV00004B/229/P